PREGNANCY GUIDE: The ultimate guide on pregnancy diet and exercise. A modern approach to understand pregnancy and successful parenting

Frances J. Lerner, 2022

Table of Contents

Chapter 1

YOU ARE PREGNANT

Pregnancy happens when a sperm fertilizes an egg after it's released from the ovary during ovulation. The fertilized egg then travels down into the uterus, where implantation happens. A successful implantation results in pregnancy.

On average, a fully Many variables may affect a pregnancy. Women who obtain an early pregnancy diagnosis and prenatal care are more likely to enjoy a healthy pregnancy and give birth to a healthy baby.

Knowing what to anticipate throughout the complete pregnant term is vital for monitoring both your health and the health of the baby.

Symptoms of pregnancy

You may notice certain signs and symptoms before you ever take a pregnancy test. Others may show weeks later, as your hormone levels alter.

Missed period

A missing menstruation is one of the early signs of pregnancy (and maybe the most typical one) (and maybe the most classic one). However, a missing period doesn't always imply you're pregnant, particularly if your cycle tends to be erratic.

There are several health issues other than pregnancy that might cause a late or missing menstruation.

Headache

Headaches are typical in early pregnancy. They're frequently caused by changed hormone levels and increased blood volume. Contact your doctor if your headaches don't go away or are very severe.

Spotting

Some women may have minor bleeding and spotting in early pregnancy. This bleeding is most typically the outcome of implantation. Implantation normally happens one to two weeks following conception.

Weight gain

You should anticipate to gain between 1 and 4 pounds in your first few months of pregnancy. Weight gain becomes more obvious at the beginning of your second trimester.

Pregnancy-induced hypertension

High blood pressure, or hypertension, sometimes occurs during pregnancy. Several variables may raise your risk, including: being overweight or obese, smoking,having a past history or a family history of pregnancy-induced hypertension.

Heartburn

Hormones produced during pregnancy may occasionally loosen the valve between your stomach and oesophagus. When stomach acid spills out, this might result in heartburn.

Constipation

Hormone changes during early pregnancy might slow down your digestive system. As a consequence, you may get constipated.

Cramps

As the muscles in your uterus begin to stretch and develop, you may experience a tugging feeling that mimics menstruation pains. If spotting or blood occurs with your cramps, it might signify a miscarriage or an ectopic pregnancy.

Back pain

Hormones and tension on the muscles are the primary causes of back discomfort in early pregnancy. Later on, your increased weight and shifting centre of gravity may contribute to your back discomfort. Around half of all pregnant women feel back discomfort throughout their pregnancy.

Anaemia

Pregnant women have an increased risk of anaemia, which produces symptoms such as lightheadedness and dizziness. The syndrome may lead to preterm delivery and low birth weight. Prenatal care frequently entails screening for anaemia.

Depression

Between 14 and 23 per cent of all pregnant women suffer depression throughout their pregnancy. The various bodily and mental changes you undergo might be significant reasons. Be careful to notify your doctor if you don't feel like your regular self.

Insomnia

Insomnia is another typical symptom of early pregnancy. Stress, physical pain, and hormonal fluctuations all be contributory reasons. A balanced diet, excellent sleep habits, and yoga stretches may all help you obtain a good night's sleep.

Breast changes

Breast changes are one of the earliest apparent indications of pregnancy. Even before you're far enough along for a positive test, your breasts may begin to feel sensitive, swollen, and generally heavy or full. Your nipples may also get bigger and more sensitive, and the areolae may darken.

Acne

Because of elevated androgen hormones, many women have acne in early pregnancy. These hormones may make your face oilier, which can block pores. Pregnancy acne is generally transient and clears up once the baby is delivered.

Vomiting

Vomiting is a component of "morning sickness," a frequent symptom that normally starts during the first four months. Morning sickness is frequently the first indicator that you're pregnant. Increased hormones during early pregnancy are the major culprit.

Hip discomfort

Hip discomfort is prevalent throughout pregnancy and tends to intensify in late pregnancy. It may have a number of reasons, including strain on your ligaments, sciatica, changes in your posture, a heavier uterus

Diarrhoea

Diarrhoea and other digestive issues occur often during pregnancy. Hormone changes, a changing diet, and additional stress are all plausible factors. If diarrhoea lasts longer than a few days, call your doctor to make sure you don't get dehydrated.

PREGNANCY TEST

A pregnancy test can establish whether a woman is pregnant. The test may be carried out at home or at the doctor's office. A pregnancy test is roughly 99 per cent accurate. It operates by monitoring levels of a hormone called human chorionic gonadotropin (HCG) (HCG). HCG may be found in the blood and urine from 10 to 14 days after pregnancy. If positive, it confirms you are pregnant.

Chapter 2

WOMEN'S WORRIES ABOUT PREGNANCY.

All pregnant women grow a bit anxiety as their due date approaches. About 20 percent of women confess that they're terrified of giving birth, and 6 to 10 percent have a birthing phobia. During a first pregnancy, it's commonly the dread of the unknown and of losing control that makes women apprehensive. For a second pregnancy, worry often originates from a poor experience the first time they gave birth. However, even if everything went perfectly the first time, there are still certain aspects of the unknown with a second or third birth that might make some women concerned.

In general, women who dread delivery are terrified of the labour pain and worry they won't be able to manage it appropriately.

They also dread losing control of their emotions. Fear might also be increased by terrible accounts of delivery they've heard from friends or family members, or by dramatic depictions seen on television.

Let's explore typical anxieties and anxiety encountered by expectant ladies;

1. The dread of giving birth, it might be good to learn about the delivery process and obtain answers to your concerns by talking to your doctor or midwife. It's an excellent time to speak about your anxieties with someone you trust. Prenatal courses are also an excellent way to become educated. Doing visualization exercises and interacting with women who've had a great experience may also help minimize the dread of giving birth. Lastly, ladies who dread delivery should bear in mind that there are no

right or wrong methods to have a kid; no matter what, they'll do their best.

2. Fear of not getting your pre-baby figure back. Some women may have anxieties about their physical appearance. They fear that they won't be beautiful anymore, that they'll gain too much weight, or that they'll lose their pre-pregnancy shape. Pregnancy is essentially a physical experience, and the anxiety of losing control over all these fast physiological changes is quite distressing for many women. It's vital to be gentle to yourself and recognize that your body will require some time to recuperate. Healthy dietary habits and physical exercise may assist.

3. Fear of being overwhelmed by mother's responsibility. Some

expecting moms may be worried of getting overwhelmed by their new position as a mother. It's common to feel this way from time to time. If you're feeling these worries, consider getting assistance throughout the first few weeks with your infant. Learning about nursing and infant care throughout your pregnancy might also help you feel more secure when the baby comes.

4. Fear of not being a good mother. Many parents fear that they won't be able to care for their kid or love them sufficiently. They may, however, take comfort in knowing that the parent-child bond will gradually grow as they spend time with their little one. In addition, the mother has already created a particular attachment with her kid over the nine months of pregnancy.

5. Fear of losing the baby or that the baby won't be healthy. This is one of the most widespread worries. Some women fear that the pregnancy isn't progressing well or that they've done something that might affect their baby's health. If the expecting woman has had a miscarriage, given birth prematurely, or had fertility issues, she may also be anxious that her body won't be able to take the baby to term. In addition, waiting for the results of medical tests done during pregnancy might make some pregnant moms more apprehensive.

Figuring out the cause of your anxieties can assist lessen anxiety. It's also crucial to bear in mind that the great majority of pregnancies conclude with the delivery of a healthy baby. To minimize anxiety, expecting moms should attempt relaxation techniques or undertake things they like to relieve tension. It's crucial to concentrate your efforts on what you can manage and let go of the rest.

Anxiety during pregnancy has been related with depressive symptoms after delivery, which is why it's so crucial to get support. In reality, anxiety symptoms typically combine with depressive symptoms. Research has revealed that roughly 18 percent of pregnant women have mild depression during pregnancy, and 7 to 12 percent of women may experience moderate to severe depression. Don't wait until you're in extreme difficulty before consulting a doctor. Early action makes it simpler to fix the issue fast and decreases the likelihood of consequences.

Chapter 3

IDEAL FOOD CONTENT FOR PREGNANT WOMEN

Pregnancy leads to substantial changes in hormone levels, it's necessary to pay attention to the food. Nutrition experts believe that mother-to-be should acquire all the important nutrients including a sufficient number of vitamins and minerals.

The following foods are good to your health and fetal growth during pregnancy:

Vegetables: carrots, sweet potatoes, pumpkin, spinach, boiled greens, tomatoes and red sweet peppers (for vitamin A and potassium)

Fruits: cantaloupe, honeydew, mangoes, prunes, bananas, apricots, oranges, and red or pink grapefruit (for potassium)

Dairy: fat-free or low-fat yogurt, skim or 1 percent milk, soymilk (for calcium, potassium, vitamins A and D)

Grains: ready-to-eat cereals/cooked cereals (for iron and folic acid)

Proteins: beans and peas; nuts and seeds; lean beef, lamb and pig; salmon, trout, herring, sardines and pollock

Foods to Avoid During Pregnancy

Avoid consuming the following items during pregnancy:

Unpasteurized milk and goods manufactured with unpasteurized milk (soft cheeses, including feta, queso blanco and fresco, Camembert, brie or blue-veined cheeses—unless labeled “made with pasteurized milk")

Hot dogs and luncheon meats (unless they are cooked till boiling hot before dishing)

Raw and undercooked seafood, eggs and meat. Do not eat sushi produced with raw fish (cooked sushi is okay) (cooked sushi is safe).

Refrigerated pâté and meat spreads

Refrigerated smoked seafood.

Prenatal Vitamin and Mineral Supplements

Most health care doctors or midwives will prescribe a prenatal vitamin before conception or soon following to make sure that all of your nutritional requirements are addressed. However, a prenatal vitamin does not substitute a balanced diet.

The Importance of Folic Acid

The U.S. Public Health Service advises that all women of reproductive age ingest 400 micrograms (0.4 mg) of folic acid each day. Folic acid is a vitamin present in:

Some green leafy veggies

Most berries, nuts, legumes, citrus fruits and fortified breakfast cereals

Some vitamin supplements.

Folic acid may help lower the chance of neural tube abnormalities, which are birth disorders of the brain and spinal cord. Neural tube abnormalities may lead to varied degrees of paralysis, incontinence and occasionally intellectual incapacity.

Chapter 4

MANAGING WEIGHT GAIN DURING PREGNANCY

Physical appearance is a priority for most women and eating healthy during pregnancy may seem tough, particularly with food cravings and aversions. It is vital to control weight gain during pregnancy.

1. **Make your desires productive**

No one expects you to skip French fries and ice cream totally while you're pregnant. After all, eating cravings come with the territory.

The goal is to fulfill your desires while receiving the protein and good fats that you and your baby need (and that will help you feel full). Make fruits your snack, fruits with

loads of fiber and high water content – like grapefruit, oranges, apples, berries, pears, and plums – may also help you feel full and keep constipation at bay. Choose a variety of colors and varieties of fruit throughout the day. Include lots of deep-pigmented berries, which give a reduced glycemic load, are a wonderful source of fiber, and are filled with phytonutrients.
"A small technique I employ is to blend something nutritious with one of my less-healthy urges," adds Largeman-Roth. "For example, I blend a high-fiber cereal with some very wonderful granola on top. You get the fiber you need to help avoid constipation, plus the delicious crunch you're seeking."

2. Choose complex carbohydrates

Carbohydrates may be a pregnant woman's greatest friend, particularly if you're suffering the nausea and vomiting of morning sickness. But simple carbohydrates such as white bread, rice, baked goods, many morning cereals, and pasta elevate your blood sugar without providing you the nutrients that comes with whole grains.

Better to reach for complex carbohydrates – such as beans, fruits and vegetables, brown rice, quinoa, and whole grain breads and pastas – which not only provide you and your baby with more nutrients, but will help you feel full for longer and make you less likely to give in to unhealthy cravings later in the day.

3. Good dehydration

It's vital to prevent dehydration during pregnancy - and drinking enough water has the extra advantage of helping you feel content between meals and snacks.

The American College of Obstetricians and Gynecologists (ACOG) encourages pregnant women to consume 8 to 12 cups (64 to 96 ounces) of water everyday. Some nutritionists advocate adding extra for each hour of mild exercise.

Other specialists propose monitoring urine color: If it's dark yellow or hazy, your body needs additional fluids. Sip throughout the day to maintain your urine color light yellow or clear — an indication of appropriate hydration.

Drinking water also eases constipation, one of the less cheerful side effects of developing a person inside of you. When you're pregnant, your digestive system slows down, which ensures that you extract every possible bit of nourishment from your meals. Getting adequate water can help keep things moving forward and also avoid painful bloating.

4. Make body weight a frequent discussion

Having a chat about weight gain with your doctor or midwife at every prenatal appointment can help you remain on track and make adjustments if you need to.

Chapter 5

SAFE EXERCISE DURING PREGNANCY

Exercise during pregnancy has several physical and mental advantages. Physical exercise may also help manage certain symptoms of pregnancy and make you feel better, knowing you're doing something healthy for yourself and your baby. As pregnancy advances, your weight will grow and you will see changes in weight distribution and body form. This leads in the body's centre of gravity shifting forward, which might impair your balance and coordination.

Some of the advantages of frequent exercise during your pregnancy include:

- enjoyment
- increased energy
- Improved fitness

- reduced back and pelvic pain
- decreased risk of pregnancy problems such as pre-eclampsia and pregnancy-induced hypertension
- preparation for the physical demands of labour
- Fewer complications in delivery
- faster recovery after labour
- prevention and management of urine incontinence
- better posture
- improved circulation
- Weight control
- stress relief
- Reduced risk of anxiety and sadness

better sleep and treatment of insomnia increased capacity to deal with the physical demands of parenthood.

Suggested fitness activities during pregnancy

Activities that are typically safe during pregnancy, especially for novices, include:

Start a short walking regimen

One of the most useful things a pregnant woman can do is walk. 10 minutes every 30 days is a decent start, for almost pregnant ladies.

- swimming
- cycling – outdoors or on a stationary bicycle
- jogging\muscle strengthening exercises, including pelvic floor exercises
- workout in water (aquarobics) (aquarobics)

yoga, stretching and other floor activities

- Pilates
- pregnancy exercise courses
- playing with pregnant ball
- resting with pregnancy pillow

Cautions for pregnant exercise

While most types of exercise are safe, there are certain workouts that entail postures and motions that may be unpleasant or hazardous for pregnant women. Be advised by your doctor or physiotherapist, but common warnings include:

Avoid elevating your body temperature too high - for example, don't bathe in hot spas or exercise to the point of excessive perspiration. Reduce your degree of exertion on hot or humid days. Stay properly hydrated.

Don't workout to the point of weariness.

If weight training, consider modest weights and medium to high repetitions - avoid lifting big weights entirely.

Perform moderate stretching and avoid over-extending.

Avoid exercising if you are unwell or feverish.

If you don't feel like exercising on a specific day, don't! It is crucial to listen to your body to prevent excessively draining your energy reserves.

Don't increase the intensity of your sports program while you are pregnant, and always work at less than 75 per cent of your maximum heart rate.

In addition, if you develop a sickness or a problem of pregnancy, discuss with your doctor or midwife before continuing or resuming your exercise regimen.

Exercises to avoid when pregnant

During pregnancy, avoid sports and activities with elevated risk of, or typified by:

- abdominal stress or pressure – such as weightlifting
- contact or collision– such as martial arts, soccer, basketball and other competitive sports
- hard projectile items or hitting instruments – such as hockey, cricket or softball
- falling – such as downhill skiing, horse riding and skating
- extreme balance, co-ordination and agility – such as gymnastics
- severe fluctuations in pressure – such as SCUBA diving

- heavy lifting

high-altitude training at above 2000 m, supine workout posture (laying on your back) – the weight of the baby may hinder the return of blood to the heart; some of these exercises can be adjusted by lying on your side, wide squats or lunges.

SUMMARY

Successful sperm implantation results in pregnancy. Knowing what to expect during the whole pregnant time is crucial for monitoring both your health and the health of the kid. Symptoms of pregnancy, pregnancy tests, and the regular anxiety and worries of pregnant women were emphasized. Pregnancy leads to substantial changes in the hormone and needs a lot of vital nutrients, to that impact, Ideal diet for pregnant women was added.

Exercise during pregnancy provides numerous physical and emotional benefits. Physical activity may also help reduce some symptoms of pregnancy and make you feel better.

Enjoy a healthy pregnancy period with this book.

www.ingramcontent.com/pod-product-compliance
Lightning Source LLC
LaVergne TN
LVHW020537160826
845677LV00015B/4107

* 9 7 9 8 8 4 6 4 1 6 8 7 1 *